Copyright ©2020 SCOTT WILSON MD.

All rights reserved. No part of this publication may be reproduced, distributed, or transmitted in any form or by any means, including photocopying, recording, or other electronic or mechanical methods, without the prior written permission of the publisher, except in the case of brief quotations embodied in critical reviews and certain other noncommercial uses permitted by copyright law.

Table of Contents

Introduction

Genital warts are an epidermal manifestation attributed to the epidermotropic human papillomavirus (HPV). More than 100 types of double-stranded HPV papovaviruses have been isolated thus far, and, of these, about 35 types have affinity to genital sites. Many have been linked directly to an increased neoplastic risk in men and women.

Two general categories of genital human papillomavirus (HPV) exist: low-risk benign HPV lesions and high-risk neoplastic HPV lesions. The low-risk strains are responsible for genital warts and recurrent respiratory papillomatosis (RRP), as well as low-grade cervical lesions. Two types, 6 and 11, account for more than 90% of genital warts and most cases of RRP. These are least likely to have malignant potential.

Thirteen human papillomavirus (HPV) types (ie, 33, 35, 39, 40, 43, 45, 51-56, 58) have a moderate risk for neoplastic conversion; HPV-16 and HPV-18 are considered high risk; more than 70% of cervical, vaginal, and penile cancers are caused from 2 types. This picture is complicated by the proven coexistence of many types in the same patient (10-15%), lack of adequate information on the oncogenic potential of many other types, and ongoing identification of additional HPV-related clinical pathology. For example, bowenoid papulosis, seborrheic keratoses, and Buschke-Lowenstein tumors —previously parts of the differential diagnosis of genital warts—all have been linked to HPV infections.

Bowenoid papulosis consists of rough papular eruptions and is considered a carcinoma in situ. Eruptions can be red, brown, or flesh colored and may regress or become invasive.

Seborrheic keratoses previously were considered a benign skin manifestation. These consist of rough plaques and have an infectious and an oncogenic potential.

Buschke-Lowenstein tumor (giant condyloma) is a fungating, locally invasive, low-grade cancer attributed to HPV.

Genital warts are soft growths that appear on the genitals. They can cause pain, discomfort, and itching.

Genital warts a sexually transmitted infection (STI) caused by certain low-risk strains of the human papillomavirus (HPV). These are different from the high-risk strains that can lead to cervical dysplasia and cancer.

HPV is the most common of all STIs. Men and women who are sexually active are vulnerable to complications of HPV, including genital warts. HPV infection is especially dangerous for women because some types of HPV can also cause cancer of the cervix and vulva.

Treatment is key in managing this infection.

Pathophysiology

Human papillomavirus (HPV) invades cells of the basal layer of the epidermis, penetrating skin and mucosal microabrasions in the genital area.

A latency period of 3 weeks to 9 months may ensue. Following that period, viral DNA, capsids, and particles are produced. Host cells become infected and develop the morphologic atypical koilocytosis of genital warts.

Most frequently affected are the penis, vulva, vagina, cervix, perineum, and perianal area. These mucosal lesions occasionally can be found in the oropharynx, larynx, and trachea. HPV-6 even has been reported in other uncommon areas (eg, extremities).

Multiple simultaneous lesions are common and may involve subclinical states as well as different anatomic sites. Subclinical infections have an infectious and oncogenic potential. However, most infections are transient and clear up within 2 years without intervention.

Consider the possibility of sexual abuse in pediatric cases; however, remember that infection by direct manual contact or, rarely, by indirect transmission from fomites may occur. Additionally, passage through an infected vaginal canal at birth may cause respiratory lesions in infants.

Etiology

Genital warts are caused by several of the epidermotropic human papillomaviruses (HPVs). HPV-6 and HPV-11 most commonly are isolated; however, many of the more than 60 types of HPV may cause condyloma. Male sex partners of women with cervical intraepithelial neoplasia often have infections of the same viral type.

Smoking, oral contraceptives, multiple sex partners, and early coital age are risk factors for acquiring genital warts.

Epidemiology

Annual incidence is 1%, and genital warts are considered the most common sexually transmitted disease (STD). A four-fold or more increase in prevalence has been reported in the last two decades; prevalence reportedly exceeds 50%. The lifetime risk of infection is 50% in sexually active individuals.

International

Reports vary on international prevalence, but available data from England, Panama, Italy, the Netherlands, and other developed and underdeveloped countries show HPV infections to be at least as common internationally as in the United States.

Sex

Both sexes are susceptible to infection. Overt disease may be more common in men (reported in 75% of cases); however, infection may be more prevalent in women.

Age

Prevalence is greatest in persons aged 17-33 years, with a peak incidence in persons aged 20-24 years.

Prognosis

Many cases of genital warts fail to respond to treatment or recur after adequate response. The recurrence rate of cervical dysplasia in women is not altered by treatment of their sex partners.

Recurrence rates exceed 50% after 1 year and have been attributed to the following:

Recurrent infection from sexual contact

Long incubation period of HPV

Location of the virus in superficial skin layers away from lymphatics

Persistence of the virus in the surrounding skin, in the hair follicle, or in sites inadequately reached by the intervention

Missed or deep lesions

Subclinical lesions

Underlying immunosuppression

Mortality is secondary to malignant transformation to a carcinoma. This oncogenic potential, which is rare with HPV-6 and HPV-11 (the most commonly isolated viruses), reportedly triples the risk of genitourinary cancer among infected males.

HPV infection appears to be more common and worse in patients with various types of immunologic deficiencies. Recurrence rate, size, discomfort, and risk of oncologic progression are highest among these patients. Secondary infection is uncommon. Latent illness often becomes active during pregnancy.

Vulvar warts may interfere with parturition. Trauma then may occur, producing crusting or erythema. Acute urethral obstruction may occur in women.

Bleeding has been reported due to flat warts of the penile urethral meatus (usually associated with HPV-16) and in the large lesions that can occur during pregnancy. Lesions may lead to disfigurement.

There is an associated psychosocial burden of external lesions on the genitalia.

Patient Education

Identify and educate persons at risk. For patient education resources, visit the Sexual Health Center. Also, see the patient education article Genital Warts.

Women's Sexual Problems

Any sexual problem that persists for more than a few weeks is worth a visit to your health care provider. He or she can rule out medical or medication causes of the problem and can offer advice on solving other types of problems.

Penis Disorders

There are two primary disorders that affect the male reproductive external organs. These include penis disorders and testicular disorders. Disorders of the penis and testes can affect a man's sexual functioning and fertility.

Sexually Transmitted Diseases

Sexually transmitted diseases, commonly called STDs, are diseases that are spread by having sex with someone who has an STD. You can get a sexually transmitted disease from sexual activity that involves the mouth, anus, vagina, or penis.

Sexual Abuse and Assault Against Women

Violence against women by any one is always wrong, whether the abuser is someone you date; a current or past spouse, boyfriend, or girlfriend; a family member; an acquaintance; or a stranger. You are not at fault

What are the symptoms of genital warts?

Genital warts are transmitted through sexual activity, including oral, vaginal, and anal sex. You may not start to develop warts for several weeks or months after infection.

Genital warts aren't always visible to the human eye. They may be very small and the color of the skin or slightly darker. The top of the growths may resemble a cauliflower and may feel smooth or slightly bumpy to the touch. They may occur as a cluster of warts, or just one wart.

Genital warts on males may appear on the following areas:

- penis

- scrotum

- groin

- thighs

- inside or around the anus

For females, these warts may appear:

- inside of the vagina or anus

- outside of the vagina or anus

- on the cervix

Genital warts may also appear on the lips, mouth, tongue, or throat of a person who has had oral sexual contact with a person who has HPV.

Even if you can't see genital warts, they may still cause symptoms, such as:

- vaginal discharge

- itching

- bleeding

- burning

If genital warts spread or become enlarged, the condition can be uncomfortable or even painful.

What causes genital warts?

Most cases of genital warts are caused by HPV. There are 30 to 40 strains of HPV that specifically affect the genitals, but just a few of these strains cause genital warts.

The HPV virus is highly transmittable through skin-to-skin contact, which is why it's considered an STI.

In fact, HPV is so common that the Centers for Disease Control and Prevention (CDC)Trusted Source says that most sexually active people get it at some point.

However, the virus doesn't always lead to complications such as genital warts. In fact, in most cases, the virus goes away on its own without causing any health problems.

Genital warts are usually caused by strains of HPV that differ from the strains that cause warts on your hands or other parts of the body. A wart can't spread from someone's hand to the genitals, and vice versa.

Risk factors for genital warts

Any sexually active person is at risk of getting HPV. However, genital warts are more common for people who:

- are under the age of 30
- smoke
- have a weakened immune system
- have a history of child abuse
- are children of a mother who had the virus during childbirth

What are other possible complications of HPV?

HPV infection is the main cause of cancer in the cervix. It can also lead to precancerous changes to the cells of the cervix, which is called dysplasia.

Other types of HPV may also cause cancer of the vulva, which are the external genital organs of women. They can also cause penile and anal cancer.

How are genital warts diagnosed?

To diagnose this condition, your doctor will ask questions about your health and sexual history. This includes symptoms you've experienced and whether you've engaged in sex, including oral sex, without condoms or oral dams.

Your doctor will also perform a physical examination of any areas where you suspect warts may be occurring.

For women only

Because warts can occur deep inside a woman's body, your doctor may need to do a pelvic examination. They may apply a mild acidic solution, which helps to make the warts more visible.

Your doctor may also do a Pap test (also known as a Pap smear), which involves taking a swab of the area to obtain cells from your cervix. These cells can then be tested for the presence of HPV.

Certain types of HPV may cause abnormal results on a Pap test, which may indicate precancerous changes. If your doctor detects these abnormalities, you may need either more frequent screenings to monitor any changes or a specialized procedure called a colposcopy.

If you're a woman and concerned that you may have contracted a form of HPV known to cause cervical cancer, your doctor can perform a DNA test. This determines what strain of HPV you have in your system. An HPV test for men isn't yet available.

How are genital warts treated?

While visible genital warts often go away with time, HPV itself can linger in your skin cells. This means you may have several outbreaks over the course of your life. So managing symptoms is important because you want to avoid transmitting the virus to others. That said, genital warts can be passed on to others even when there are no visible warts or other symptoms.

You may wish to treat genital warts to relieve painful symptoms or to minimize their appearance. However, you can't treat genital warts with over-the-counter (OTC) wart removers or treatments.

Your doctor may prescribe topical wart treatments that might include:

- imiquimod (Aldara)
- podophyllin and podofilox (Condylox)
- trichloroacetic acid, or TCA

If visible warts don't go away with time, you may need minor surgery to remove them. Your doctor can also remove the warts through these procedures:

- electrocautery, or burning warts with electric currents
- cryosurgery, or freezing warts
- laser treatments
- excision, or cutting off warts
- injections of the drug interferon

Home remedies for genital warts

Don't use OTC treatments meant for hand warts on genital warts. Hand and genital warts are caused by different strains of HPV, and treatments designed for other areas of the body are often much stronger than treatments used on the genitals. Using the wrong treatments may do more harm than good.

Some home remedies are touted as helpful in treating genital warts, but there is little evidence to support them.

Always check with your doctor before trying a home remedy.

How to prevent genital warts

HPV vaccines called Gardasil and Gardasil 9 can protect men and women from the most common HPV strains that cause genital warts, and can also protect against strains of HPV that are linked to cervical cancer.

A vaccine called Cervarix is also available. This vaccine protects against cervical cancer, but not against genital warts.

Individuals up to age 45 years can receive the HPV vaccine, as well as those as young as age 9. The vaccine is administered in a series of two or three shots, depending on age. Both types of vaccine should be given before the person becomes sexually active, as they're most effective before a person is exposed to HPV.

Using a condom or a dental dam every time you have sex can also reduce your risk of contracting genital warts.

The important thing is to use a physical barrier to prevent transmission.

Coping and outlook

Genital warts are a complication of HPV infection that's common and treatable. They can disappear over time, but treatment is essential in preventing their return and possible complications.

If you think you have genital warts, talk to your doctor. They can determine if you have warts and what your best treatment options are.

In addition, it's important to talk to your sexual partner. This may sound difficult, but being open about your condition can help you protect your partner from also getting an HPV infection and genital warts.

What happens at a sexual health clinic

A doctor or nurse can usually diagnose warts by looking at them.

They will:

- ask you about your symptoms and sexual partners
- look at the bumps around your genitals and anus, maybe using a magnifying lens
- possibly need to look inside your vagina, anus or urethra (where pee comes out), depending on where the warts are
- It may not be possible to find out who you got genital warts from, or how long you've had the infection.

Treatment for genital warts

Treatment for genital warts needs to be prescribed by a doctor.

The type of treatment you'll be offered depends on what the warts look like and where they are. The doctor or nurse will discuss this with you.

Treatments include:

- cream or liquid: you can usually apply this to the warts yourself a few times a week for several weeks, but in some cases you may need to go to a sexual health clinic where a doctor or nurse will apply it. These treatments can cause pain, irritation or a burning sensation.

- surgery: a doctor or nurse may cut, burn or use a laser to remove the warts. This can cause pain, irritation or scarring.

- freezing: a doctor or nurse freezes the warts. Sometimes the treatment is repeated several times. This can cause pain.

- It may take weeks or months for treatment to work and the warts may come back. In some people, the treatment does not work.

There's no cure for genital warts, but it's possible for your body to fight the virus over time.

Do

- tell the doctor or nurse if you're pregnant or thinking of becoming pregnant, as some treatments will not be suitable for you

- avoid perfumed soap, shower gel or bath products during treatment because these can irritate your skin

- ask the doctor or nurse if your treatment will affect condoms, diaphragms or caps

Don't

- do not use wart treatment from a pharmacy; these are not made for genital warts

- do not smoke; many treatments for genital warts work better if you do not smoke

- do not have vaginal, anal or oral sex until the warts have gone; but if you do have sex, always use a condom

How genital warts are passed on

- The genital warts virus can be passed on even when there are no visible warts.

- Many people with the virus do not have symptoms but can still pass it on.

- If you have genital warts, your current sexual partners should get tested because they may have warts and not know it.

- After you get the infection, it can take weeks to many months before symptoms appear.

You can get genital warts from:

- skin-to-skin contact, including vaginal and anal sex
- sharing sex toys
- oral sex, but this is rare

The virus can also be passed to a baby from its mother during birth, but this is rare.

You cannot get genital warts from:

- kissing
- sharing things like towels, cutlery, cups or toilet seats
- How to stop genital warts being passed on
- You can stop genital warts from being passed on by:
- using a condom every time you have vaginal, anal or oral sex – but if the virus is in any in skin that's not protected by a condom, it can still be passed on
- not having sex while you're having treatment for genital warts
- not sharing sex toys; if you do share them, wash them or cover them with a new condom before anyone else uses them

Why genital warts come back

Genital warts are caused by a virus called human papillomavirus (HPV). There are many types of HPV.

The HPV virus can stay in your skin and warts can develop again.

Warts may go away without treatment, but this may take many months. You can still pass the virus on, and the warts may come back.

Genital warts and cancer

Genital warts are not cancer and do not cause cancer.

The HPV vaccine that's offered to girls and boys aged 12 to 13 in England protects against cervical cancer and genital warts.

The HPV vaccine is also offered to men (up to the age of 45) who have sex with men (MSM), some trans men and trans women, sex workers, and men and women living with HIV.

Genital warts and pregnancy

Important

Tell your midwife or doctor if:

you're pregnant, or think you're pregnant, and you have genital warts or think you have genital warts

During pregnancy, genital warts:

- can grow and multiply
- might appear for the first time, or come back after a long time of not being there
- can be treated safely, but some treatments should be avoided
- may be removed if they're very big, to avoid problems during birth
- may be passed to the baby during birth, but this is rare; the HPV virus can cause infection in the baby's throat or genitals

Most pregnant women with genital warts have a vaginal delivery. Very rarely you might be offered a caesarean, depending on your circumstances.

How Do People Get Genital Warts?

The HPV that causes genital warts usually spreads through vaginal, oral, or anal sex or close sexual contact with the genital area. Even if there are no warts, HPV might still be active in the genital area and can spread to others.

It is not always possible for people to know when they got infected with HPV. This is because:

the virus can be in the body for months to years before warts develop

they might have had warts before that weren't noticed

How Long Do Genital Warts Last?

How long genital warts last can vary from person to person. Sometimes, the immune system clears the warts within a few months. But even if the warts go away, the HPV might still be active in the body. So the warts can come back. Usually within 2 years, the warts and the HPV are gone from the body.

When Is Someone With Genital Warts No Longer Contagious?

People with genital warts definitely can spread HPV. But even after the warts are gone, HPV might still be active in the body. That means it can spread to someone else through sex or close sexual contact and cause warts in that person. It's hard to know when people are no longer contagious, because there's no blood test that looks for HPV.

Most of the time, HPV is gone within 2 years of when someone was infected.

Can Genital Warts Be Prevented?

Genital warts and other types of HPV can be prevented by a vaccine. The HPV vaccine series is recommended for all kids when they're 11–12 years old. Older teens and adults also can get the vaccine (up to age 45). Even if someone already has had one type of HPV infection, the HPV vaccine can protect against other types of HPV.

HPV almost always spreads through sex. So the best way to prevent it is to not have sex (vaginal, oral, or anal). If someone does decide to have sex, using a condom every time for sex (vaginal, oral, anal) helps prevent HPV and other STDs. But condoms can't always prevent HPV because they don't cover all areas where HPV can live.

Should Sexual Partners Be Told About Genital Warts?

Someone diagnosed with genital warts should have an honest conversation with sexual partners. Partners need to be seen by a health care provider who can check for genital warts and do screenings for other STDs.

If the couple plan to continue having sex, both people need to understand that a condom will help lower the risk of spreading genital warts/HPV but can't completely prevent it.

Looking Ahead

If you or someone you know has been diagnosed with genital warts, it is important to:

- Know that HPV can spread to partners during sex, even if there are no warts.
- Tell any sexual partners about the warts before having sex.
- Use a condom every time they have sex (vaginal, oral, or anal).
- Get tested for other STDs as recommended by your health care provider.
- Gets all doses of the HPV vaccine.

What Is HPV and Why Is It a Problem?

Human papillomavirus (HPV) is one of the most common sexually transmitted diseases (STDs). HPV is the virus that causes genital warts.

Besides genital warts, an HPV infection can cause these other problems:

- In females, it can cause problems with the that may lead to cervical cancer. HPV infection also can lead to cancer in the vagina, vulva, anus, mouth, and throat.

- In males, HPV infection may lead to cancer in the penis, anus, mouth, and throat.

- New research suggests that HPV may be linked to heart disease in women.

- Both girls and guys can get HPV from sexual contact, including vaginal, oral, and anal sex. Most people infected with HPV don't know they have it because they don't notice any signs or problems. People do not always get genital warts, but the virus is still in their system and could cause damage. This means that people with HPV can pass the infection to others without knowing it.

- Because HPV can cause problems like genital warts and some kinds of cancer, a vaccine is an important step in preventing infection and protecting against the spread of HPV.

- That's why doctors recommend that all girls and guys get the vaccine from age 11 or 12 through age 26. If needed, kids can get the vaccine starting at age 9.

How Does the HPV Vaccine Work?

The HPV vaccine is recommended for people 9 to 26 years old:

- For kids and teens ages 9–14, the vaccine is given in 2 shots over a 6- to 12-month period.

- For teens and young adults (ages 15–26), it's given in 3 shots over a 6-month period.

- It works best when people get all their shots on time. If you're under age 26 and you've missed a shot, you can still catch up. Just ask your doctor about the best way to do that.

- The vaccine does not protect people against strains of HPV that might have infected them before getting the vaccine. The most effective way to prevent HPV infection is to get vaccinated before having sex for the first time. But even if you have had sex, don't give up on getting the vaccine. It's still the best way to protect against strains of the virus that you may not have come in contact with.

- The vaccine doesn't protect against all types of HPV. Anyone having sex should get routine checkups at a doctor's office or health clinic. Girls should get Pap smears when a doctor recommends it — usually around age 21 unless there are signs of a problem before that.

- The HPV vaccine is not a replacement for using condoms to protect against other strains of HPV — and other STDs — when having sex.

What Are the Side Effects of the HPV Vaccine?

Side effects that people get from the HPV vaccine usually are minor. They may include swelling or pain at the injection site, or feeling faint after getting the vaccine. As with other vaccines, there is a small chance of an allergic reaction.

A few people have reported health problems after getting the shot. The FDA is monitoring the vaccine closely to make sure these are not caused by the vaccine itself.

Most people have no trouble with the vaccine. You can make fainting less likely by sitting down for 15 minutes after each shot.

How Can I Protect Myself From HPV?

For people who have sex, condoms offer some protection against HPV. Condoms can't completely prevent infections because hard-to-see warts can be outside the area covered by a condom, and the virus can infect people even when a partner doesn't have warts. Also, condoms can break.

The only way to be completely sure about preventing HPV infections and other STDs is not to have sex (abstinence). Spermicidal foams, creams, and jellies aren't proven to protect against HPV or genital warts.

If you have questions about the vaccine or are worried about STDs, talk to your doctor.

Can You Still Get Genital Warts If You've Had All the HPV Shots?

There is a small chance that someone might still get genital warts after having all their HPV vaccine shots. The vaccine protects against 90% of the HPV strains that cause genital warts. But there are lots of different strains (types) of HPV and the vaccine cannot protect against them all.

The real purpose of the HPV vaccine is to protect against cervical and other types of cancers. Experts have found that certain strains of HPV may cause cancers of the cervix, vagina, vulva, penis, anus, mouth, and throat. The shots are designed to vaccinate people against the strains of HPV that are most likely to cause cancer.

So, like most things in life, the HPV vaccine doesn't come with a 100% guarantee. But it's still a good idea to get all the shots: When it comes to cancer, the more protected you are, the better.

Also, if you're having sex, it's still important to see your gynecologist regularly and use condoms to protect against STDs (including those strains of HPV that aren't covered by the shot).

History

Painless bumps, pruritus, and discharge are the chief complaints encountered with genital warts. Generally, two thirds of individuals who have sexual contact with a partner who has genital warts develop lesions within 3 months. A history involving multiple lesions, rather than a single isolated wart, is more common. Involvement of more than one area is more common.

History may indicate previous or other current sexually transmitted diseases (STDs). Oral, laryngeal, or tracheal mucosal lesions (uncommon) presumably transfer through oral-genital contact. History of anal intercourse warrants a thorough search for perianal lesions.

Urethral bleeding or urinary obstruction (uncommon) may be the presenting complaint when the wart involves the meatus.

Vaginal bleeding during pregnancy may be due to condyloma eruptions. Coital bleeding also may occur.

Latent illness may become active, particularly with pregnancy and immunosuppression.

Lesions may regress spontaneously, remain static, or progress.

Physical Examination

Single or multiple papular eruptions may be seen. Eruptions can be pearly, filiform, fungating, cauliflower, or plaquelike.

Lesions can be quite smooth (particularly on the penile shaft), verrucous, or lobulated. Some appear harmless, others have a more disturbing appearance. Multiple sites often are involved simultaneously.

Color may vary from that of the skin to erythema or hyperpigmentation.

Check for irregularities in shape, form, or color that may suggest melanoma or malignancy.

Seek perianal lesions, particularly in patients with a history or risk of immunosuppression or anal intercourse.

Search for evidence of other STDs (eg, ulcerations, adenopathy, vesicles, discharge).

Genital warts have a propensity for the penile glans and shaft in men and for the vulvovaginal and cervical areas in women.

Urethral meatus and mucosal lesions can occur.

Some lesions are subclinical, and some are hidden by hair or in the inner aspect of uncircumcised foreskin.

Although earlier reports have suggested otherwise, the presence of external genital warts warrants a thorough search for cervical and urethral lesions. Such internal lesions have been found in more than half of females with external lesions. Infected males have a 20% chance or more (in one report) of having subclinical urethral lesions. More than 50% of female patients with external lesions have negative Papanicolaou test (Pap smear) results but positive HPV infection results using in situ hybridization.

Pruritus may be a complaint. Discharge may be evident.

Complications

- Possible complications are as follows:
- Local disfigurement
- Transformation to genitourinary malignancies in both males and females
- Transmission to neonate or partners

Recurrence: According to Diamantis et al, recurrence rates for anogenital warts ranged from 19% at 3 months to 23% at 6 months.

Differential Diagnoses

- Condyloma Acuminatum (Genital Warts)
- Condyloma Lata (Secondary syphilis)
- Familial Benign Pemphigus (Hailey-Hailey Disease)
- Herpes Simplex
- Keratosis Follicularis (Darier Disease)
- Neoplasia

- Nevi

- Pearly Penile Papules

- Vulvar neurofibromatosis

- Vulvar vestibular papillae

Approach Considerations

As indicated by history and physical examination, consider testing for other STDs (eg, HIV, gonorrhea, chlamydia, syphilis).

The following are to assist in the understanding and management of potential complications:

Pap smear - Used to look for papillomatosis, acanthosis, koilocytic abnormality, and mild nuclear abnormality

Colposcopy (stereoscopic microscopy) - Used to look for papillomatosis, acanthosis, koilocytic abnormality, and mild nuclear abnormality

Biopsy - Indicated for lesions that are atypical, recurrent after initial success, or resistant to treatment and in patients with a high risk for neoplasia or immunosuppression

Filter hybridization (Southern blot and slot-blot hybridization), in situ hybridization, and polymerase chain reaction - Used for diagnosis and typing of HPV

Hybrid capture

Approach Considerations

Symptomatic treatment may be warranted in emergency situations. Use pressure to stop bleeding, if present. Relieve urethral obstruction (rare). Search for evidence of coexistent STDs; treat them if found and indicated. Further treatment, screening, and vaccination guidelines from the American College of Obstetricians and Gynecologists and Centers for Disease Control and Prevention are available. .

Untreated

If visible genital warts are left untreated, they can undergo spontaneous resolution, increase in size, increase in number, or remain unchanged. Complete resolution of lesions after 2 years occurs in 75% of individuals without intervention.

Ablative therapy

Cryotherapy can be used. Use an open spray or cotton-tipped applicator for 10-15 seconds and repeat as needed. Lift away mobile skin from the underlying normal tissue before freezing. Response rates are high, clearance occurs about 75% of the time with few adverse sequelae. Adverse reactions include pain during treatment, erosion, ulceration, and postinflammatory hypopigmentation of skin. Cryotherapy is safe for use during pregnancy.

Electrodesiccation (smoke plume may be infective) and curettage have been used.

Surgical excision has the highest success rate and lowest recurrence rate. Initial cure rates are 63-91%.

Carbon dioxide laser treatment is used for extensive or recurrent genital warts. The procedure requires local, regional, or general anesthesia. (A eutectic mixture of local anesthetics [EMLA] cream may be used as an alternative anesthetic.) Clearance rates are more than 90%, but reoccurrence can be up to 40%. HPV-6 DNA has been detected in the carbon dioxide laser plume; therefore, the laser operator is at risk of developing mucosal warts.

With infrared coagulation, a beam of infrared light is delivered to the affected lesions, causing tissue coagulation and necrosis. Treatment is successful in about 80% of cases.

Immune-based therapy
Physician administered treatments include acid applications (bichloroacetic acid or trichloroacetic acid) and interferon injections with antiviral mechanisms.

Medications for home use include imiquimod 5% cream, podofilox gel or solution, and antiproliferative compounds (5-fluorouracil).

Vaccination

The 9-valent HPV vaccine (Gardasil 9 [9vHPV]) is available in the United States to decrease the risk of certain cancers and precancerous lesions in males and females. The 9vHPV vaccine covers HPV subtypes 6, 11, 16, 18, 31, 33, 45, 52, and 58. Cervarix (2vHPV) and Gardasil (4vHPV) were discontinued in the United States in October 2016. Children and adolescents aged 15 years and younger need two, not three, doses of the 9vHPV vaccine; this Advisory Committee on Immunization Practices (ACIP) recommendation stems from the vaccine's enhanced immunogenicity in preteens and adolescents aged 9-14 years. The schedule for older adolescents and young adults aged 15-45 years is three inoculations within 6 months.

Approval for adults up to age 45 years was based on a study of approximately 3200 women aged 27-45 years followed for an average of 3.5 years. The 9vHPV vaccine was 88% effective in preventing the combined endpoint of persistent infection, genital warts, vulvar and vaginal precancerous lesions, cervical precancerous lesions, and cervical cancer related to HPV types covered by the vaccine.

The effectiveness of 9vHPV in men aged 27-45 years is inferred from the data described above in women, as well as from efficacy data in younger men (aged 16-26 y) and immunogenicity data from a clinical trial in which 150 men, aged 27-45 years, received a three-dose regimen over 6 months.

Special concerns
Pregnancy

Latent infections may become activated with numerous large lesions. Lesions often present or increase during pregnancy. Lesions may make vaginal delivery difficult if they are in the cervix, vagina, or vulva. Lesions tend to bleed easily. Lesions often regress spontaneously after delivery.

Pediatrics

Neonates may become infected during passage through an infected birth canal. The incidence of perinatal transmission to the infant pharynx may be as high as 50%; transmission occurs most frequently with HPV-6 and HPV-11. Incidence of genital infection in neonates is 4%, although the American College of Obstetrics and Gynecology currently does not recommend cesarean delivery due solely to positive HPV status.

Consultations

No emergent consultation is indicated. Outpatient follow-up with a dermatologist, an OB/GYN, or a urologist is indicated.

Prevention

The 9-valent HPV vaccine (Gardasil 9 [9vHPV]) is available in the United States to decrease the risk of certain cancers and precancerous lesions in males and females. 9vHPV vaccine covers HPV subtypes 6, 11, 16, 18, 31, 33, 45, 52, and 58. Cervarix (2vHPV) and Gardasil (4vHPV) were discontinued in the United States in October 2016. Children and adolescents aged 15 years and younger need two, not three, doses of the 9vHPV vaccine; this ACIP recommendation stems from the vaccine's enhanced immunogenicity in preteens and adolescents aged 9-14 years. The schedule for older adolescents and young adults aged 15 through 45 years is three inoculations within 6 months.

Approval for adults up to 45 years old was based on a study of approximately 3200 women aged between 27 through 45 years followed for an average of 3.5 years. 9vHPV vaccine was 88% effective in preventing the combined endpoint of persistent infection, genital warts, vulvar and vaginal precancerous lesions, cervical precancerous lesions, and cervical cancer related to HPV types covered by the vaccine.

Effectiveness of 9vHPV in men aged 27 through 45 years is inferred from the data described above in women, as well as efficacy data in younger men (aged 16 through 26 years) and immunogenicity data from a clinical trial in which 150 men, aged 27 through 45 years, received a 3-dose regimen over 6 months. [

Long-Term Monitoring

Ensure follow-up with a dermatologist, OB/GYN (females), or urologist (males) within 1 week. Perform a workup for human papillomavirus (HPV) and other sexually transmitted diseases (STDs) as indicated. Treat the patient using medications; if medications are ineffective, treat with cryotherapy, curettage, electrodesiccation, surgical excision, carbon dioxide laser treatment, or combination therapy.

Evaluate and treat sexual partner(s).

Search for immunosuppression in patients with treatment failures and recurrences. Perform a tissue biopsy if recurrences or treatment failures occur.

Medication Summary

Warts generally regress spontaneously within months or years. Remove genital or laryngeal warts, however, because of the possibility of malignant transformation.

The CDC recommends keratolytic agents, antimitotic agents, and immune-response modifiers as alternative regimens to cryotherapy to treat external genital/perianal warts, vaginal warts, and urethral meatus warts.

Podofilox (purified podophyllotoxin) is available for home use by the patient. A 0.5% solution is applied twice daily for 3 consecutive days followed by 4 days of no therapy. The cycle can be repeated up to 4 times. Slightly higher cure rates are expected than with podophyllin. Podofilox is useful for prophylaxis. Podofilox is not recommended as the sole treatment for recurrent warts.

Imiquimod (Aldara) 5% cream is applied qhs, 3 times a week for a treatment period of 16 weeks. The treatment area should be washed with soap and water 6-10 hours after application. Diamantis et al note that complete clearance of warts occurred in 50% of patients treated with imiquimod 5% cream (administered once-daily, 3 times/wk, up to 16 wk).

Keratolytics

Class Summary

These agents cause the cornified epithelium to swell, soften, macerate, and then desquamate.

Podophyllum resin (Podocon-25, Podo-Ben-25, Podofin)

Podophyllum resin is a powdered mixture of resins removed from the May apple (mandrake) (Podophyllum peltatum linne). It is cytotoxic agent used topically to treat genital warts. Arrests mitosis in metaphase, an effect it shares with other cytotoxic agents (eg, vinca alkaloids). Podophyllotoxin is the active agent, and its strength varies with the type of podophyllum resin used. American podophyllum contains a fourth the amount of Indian sources. A cure rate of 20-50% can be expected if used as a single agent. Clearance rates are much higher if cryotherapy is used simultaneously.

Podofilox (Condylox)

Podofilox is a topical antimitotic that can be chemically synthesized or purified from plant families Coniferae and Berberidaceae (eg, species of Juniperus and Podophyllum). Treatment of anogenital warts results in necrosis of visible wart tissue. The exact mechanism of action is unknown. Genital warts are epidemiologically associated with cervical carcinoma. Slightly higher cure rates can be expected with podofilox than with podophyllin. Additionally, this agent is useful for prophylaxis.

Trichloroacetic acid topical (Tri-Chlor)

Trichloroacetic acid topical cauterizes skin, keratin, and other tissues. Although caustic, it causes less local irritation and systemic toxicity than other agents in the same class. However, the response is often incomplete and recurrences are frequent.

5-Fluorouracil (Efudex, Fluoroplex)

5-Fluorouracil has antimetabolic, antineoplastic, and immunostimulative activity. It is useful to prevent recurrence in patients who are immunocompromised if started within 4 weeks of condyloma ablation. Mild local discomfort can be treated with cortisol cream.

Miscellaneous topical ointment

Class Summary

Another topical product that has gained FDA approval for genital warts includes kunecatechins.

Kunecatechins (Veregen)

Kunecatechins is a botanical drug product for topical use consisting of extract from green tea leaves. Its mode of action is unknown, but it does elicit antioxidant activity in vitro. It is indicated for topical treatment of external genital and perianal warts (condylomata acuminatum) in immunocompetent patients.

Interferons

Class Summary

These agents are naturally produced proteins with antiviral, antitumor, and immunomodulatory actions.

Alpha-, beta-, and gamma-interferons exist and may be administered topically, systemically, and intralesionally.

Interferon alfa-n3 (Alferon N)

Interferon alfa-n3 is approved by the FDA for injection in refractory condyloma acuminata. The mechanism by which interferons exert antitumor activity is poorly understood. Direct antiproliferative action against tumor cells and modulation of the host immune response may play important roles.

The recurrence rate is 20-40%, but the recurrence rate after successful treatment is lower than with other treatment modalities. Nevertheless, intralesional interferon is expensive and requires repeated office visits.

Immune response modifiers

Class Summary

These agents are indicated for treatment of genital warts. Induces secretion of interferon alpha and other cytokines; mechanisms of action are unknown. They may be more effective in women than in men.

Imiquimod (Aldara) 5% cream

Imiquimod induces secretion of interferon alpha and other cytokines; the mechanisms of action are unknown.

Vaccines

Class Summary

The 9-valent HPV vaccine is indicated for prevention of HPV-associated dysplasias and neoplasia, including cervical cancer, genital warts (condyloma acuminata), and precancerous genital lesions.

Children and adolescents aged 15 years and younger need two, not three, doses of the HPV vaccine; this ACIP recommendation stems from the vaccine's enhanced immunogenicity in preteens and adolescents aged 9-14 years. The schedule for older adolescents and adults aged 15-45 years is three inoculations within 6 months.

Human papillomavirus vaccine, nonavalent (Gardasil 9)

This vaccine induces a humoral immune response to 9 HPV subtypes: 6, 11, 16, 18, 31, 33, 45, 52, and 58. It is indicated in males and females aged 9-45 years to prevent HPV-associated diseases.

www.ingramcontent.com/pod-product-compliance
Lightning Source LLC
Chambersburg PA
CBHW051356150726
48000CB00003B/1215